Everything You Need to Know About Juvenile Arthritis

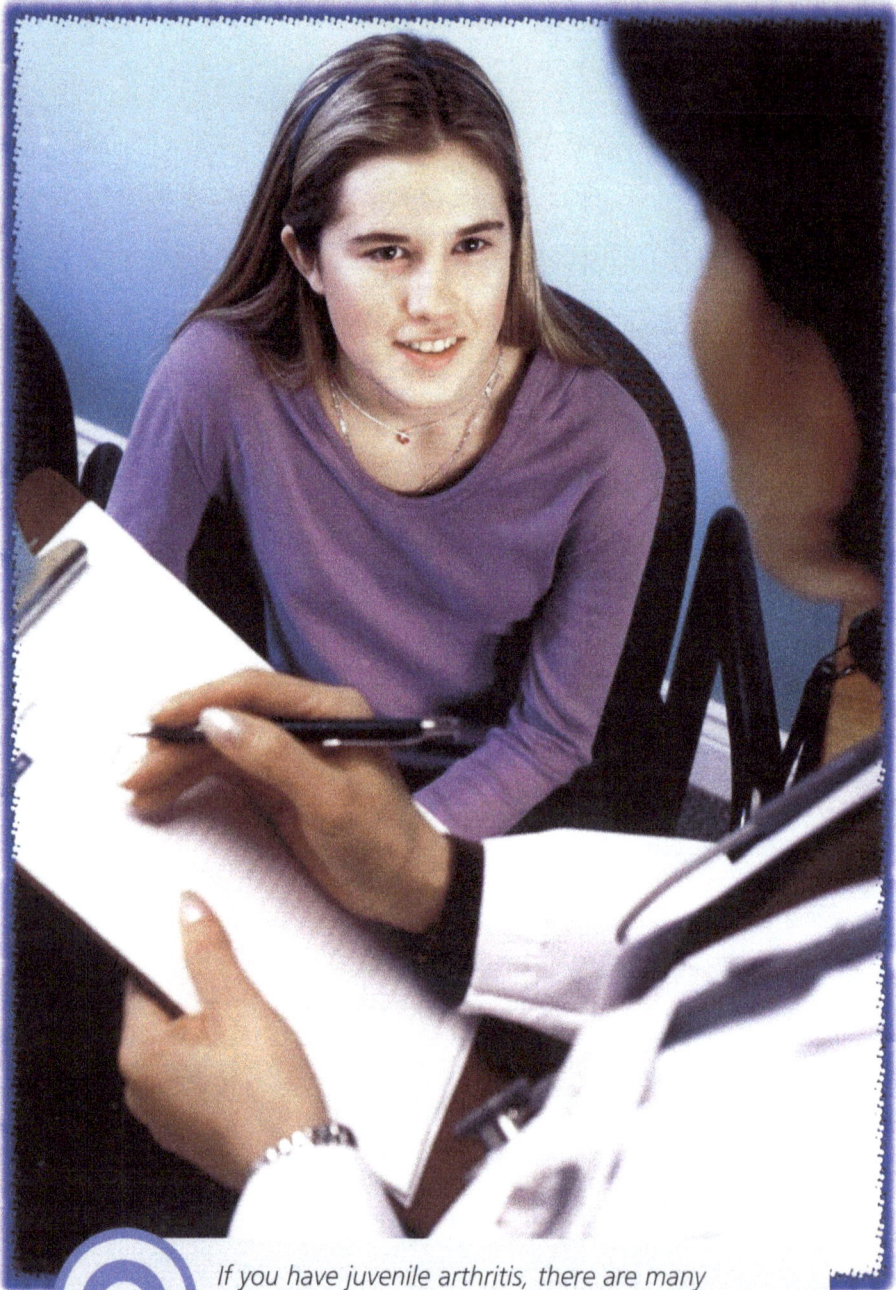

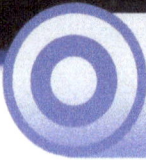

If you have juvenile arthritis, there are many opportunities for you to take an active role in your own treatment.

Everything You Need to Know About *Juvenile Arthritis*

Guy Fall

The Rosen Publishing Group, Inc.
New York

To Amelia Tereza Santa Rosa Maraux

Published in 2003 by The Rosen Publishing Group, Inc.
29 East 21st Street, New York, NY 10010

First Edition

Library of Congress Cataloging-in-Publication Data

Fall, Guy.
Everything you need to know about juvenile arthritis / by Guy Fall.
   p. cm. -- (The need to know library)
Includes bibliographical references and index.
ISBN 13: 978-1-4358-8890-6
1. Rheumatoid arthritis in children--Juvenile literature.
[1. Arthritis. 2. Diseases.]
I. Title: Juvenile arthritis. II. Title. III. Series.
RJ482.A77 F35 2002
618.92'7227--dc21

2001007995

Manufactured in the United States of America

Contents

Introduction

One spring day, I was playing soccer with some of my friends. I must have been twelve at the time. At one point, I tripped and fell. When I got up, my ankle was really sore. It started to swell, and soon it was bigger than an apple. I couldn't play anymore. In fact, I was in so much pain I couldn't walk. Crying, I called my dad and asked him to pick me up. At the hospital, X rays indicated that there was no fracture. The doctor bandaged my ankle, gave me some pills for the pain, and told me to stay off my left leg.

A month later, my ankle was still the same size, and X rays still showed nothing. Even though I was wearing special lace-up boots, my left leg hurt when I walked. The pain was so bad that I had to keep sneaking painkillers from my parents' medicine cabinet. When the pills ran out, I didn't want them to think anything was wrong, so I spent a lot of time in my room.

School was hard, though. After a while, my ankle got better, but then, my wrists, elbows, and fingers started to swell up, and they became red and sore. I hid my hands beneath long shirt-sleeves. Sometimes, in the mornings, they were so stiff I could barely move them.

My friends noticed, but when they asked me questions, I just brushed them off. Truthfully, though, I was terrified that something horrible was happening to my body.

Obviously, I couldn't go on pretending that nothing was wrong. One day, I came home from school and my parents were waiting for me with worried expressions on their faces. My homeroom teacher had called them. She had noticed that my writing was suffering and that I was having trouble getting my homework done. "You should have come to us with your pain," said my dad, looking at my swollen hands. "We need to see a doctor."

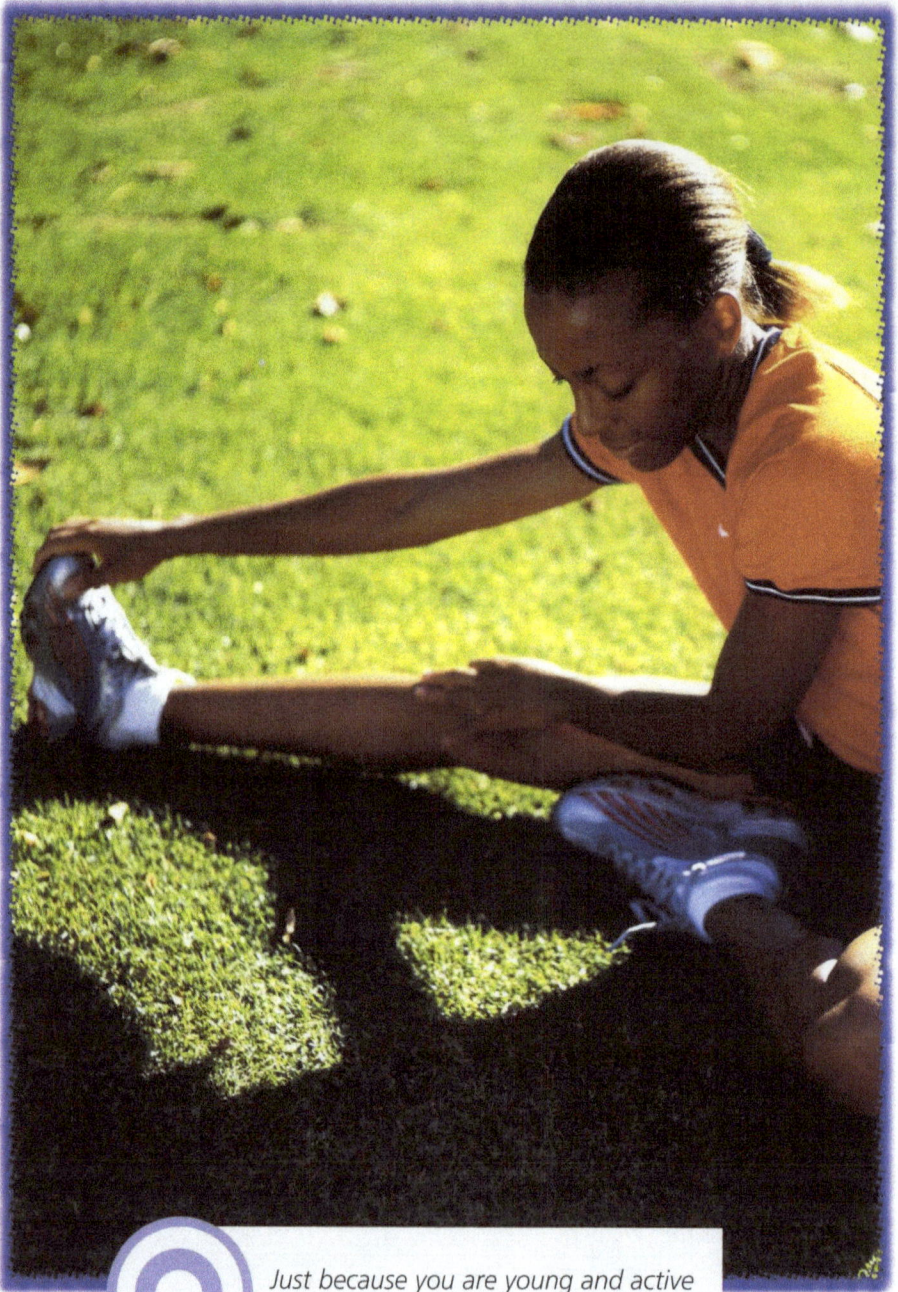

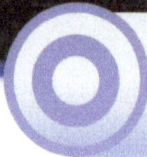

Just because you are young and active doesn't mean you can't get arthritis.

That same day, we went to the hospital and saw the doctor we had seen months before for my ankle. He examined me carefully and asked me a lot of questions. "We'll have to do some more tests and it will take a little while," he said. "But your pain and swollen joints indicate that you have a type of juvenile rheumatoid arthritis."

Both my parents and I looked at each other. We knew that our lives were going to change.

—Miranda

Many people continue to believe that arthritis is an elderly person's disease. Yet, in its various forms, juvenile rheumatoid arthritis—or JRA—affects close to 300,000 young people in the United States alone. The bad news is that nobody knows exactly what causes it. And unfortunately, there is no known cure for it. The good news is that it is increasingly possible for young people with JRA to live full lives. Proper medical attention and new drugs and medicines coupled with physical therapy are controlling JRA like never before. Meanwhile, increasing awareness of and support for arthritic youths at school and home, and the increase of JRA support groups have helped give a lot of young people the courage and determination to fight the disease—and win.

Chapter 1

Not Just an Elderly Person's Disease

Juvenile rheumatoid arthritis—aside from the "juvenile" part, it sounds like a disease that someone gets when they are around the age of seventy-five. That's because as people grow older, many of them do develop types of rheumatism and/or arthritis, and those are the cases that we are most familiar with. Both diseases are similar. Arthritis causes inflammation of the body's joints ("arthro" comes from the Greek word indicating "joints"). Rheumatism affects not only joints but also muscles, tendons, bones, and nerves, causing discomfort and disability.

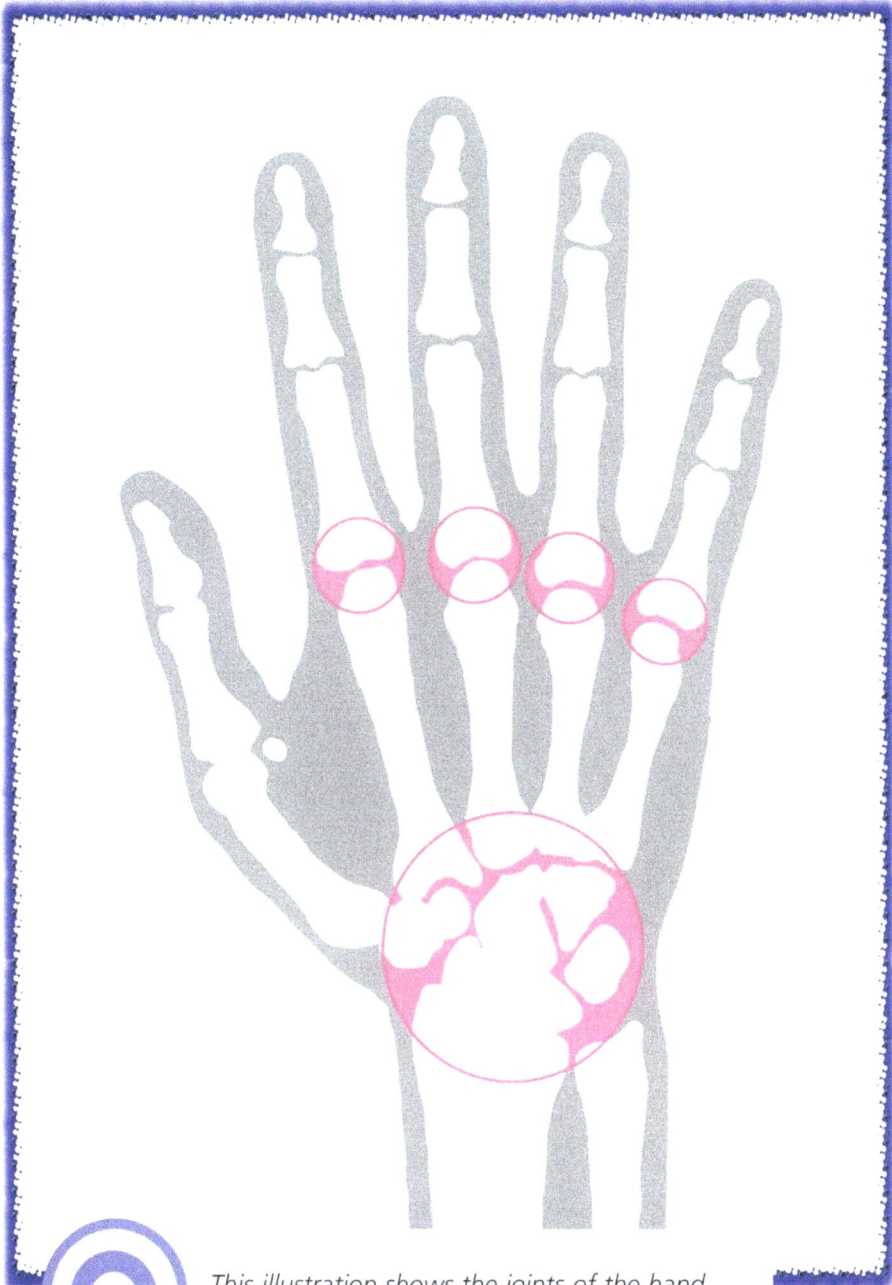

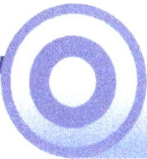

This illustration shows the joints of the hand (in pink) that can be affected by arthritis.

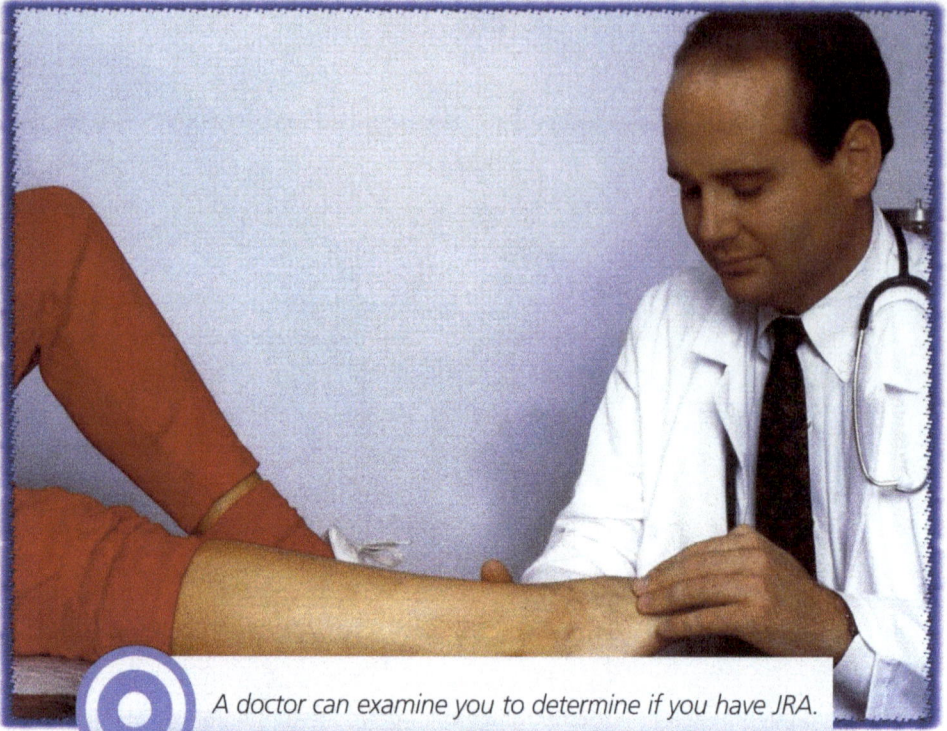

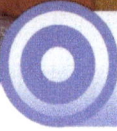

A doctor can examine you to determine if you have JRA.

What Is JRA?

Inflammation occurs when a body part—such as a joint or muscle—swells up, becoming hot, reddish in color, and painful. Young people under the age of sixteen who experience arthritis in their joints for longer than six weeks likely have JRA. JRA can affect any of the body's joints. A joint is the meeting point of two bones that allows movement. The joints most commonly affected by JRA are in the fingers, wrists, elbows, shoulders, ankles, and knees.

This disease is chronic, which means that it is a continuous, long-term condition. However, most people with JRA don't live in constant pain, unable to move. In general, JRA alternates between flares and remissions. Flares can come along at any time and suddenly attack joints. Aside from dealing with pain and stiffness, motion can be very difficult. Even tasks as seemingly easy as walking down stairs or gripping a pencil can prove impossible during a flare.

When a flare is over and the body is able to function normally, the JRA has gone into remission. Remission can last for weeks, months, or even years. In fact, some young people who have JRA as kids or teens grow into adulthood and never experience a flare again. However, when flares are frequent and severe, the damage inflicted upon joints and other body parts can be serious, even to the point of permanently limiting motion.

Causes of JRA

Nobody knows what causes juvenile arthritis. It is believed that children whose parents or grandparents have some form of arthritis have slightly higher chances of acquiring JRA. However, at the same time, if one child develops JRA, it is extremely rare that a brother or sister will have it, too. To date, nobody has proved that arthritis is hereditary.

Other theories revolve around defective immune, or defense, systems. Normally, the immune system fights infections and viruses, attacking foreign invaders. In the case of JRA, however, instead of attacking substances from outside the body, the immune system reacts against the body's own healthy tissues. For this reason, JRA is known as an autoimmune disease. Autoimmune diseases occur when the immune system attacks itself.

Although the cause remains a mystery, certain events have been known to bring on initial or subsequent flares of the disease. One triggering factor can be severe stress. Severe stress can be caused by the death of a family member or close friend, an illness in the family, or the divorce or separation of one's parents, for example. Another factor can be a serious injury. One teenage boy developed JRA after falling out of a tree. Although he didn't break any bones, he developed severe arthritis in many of his joints at the moment of impact. He continued to suffer from JRA for four years.

Three Types of JRA

There are three main types of JRA. The onset of the disease—how it first reveals itself in its early stages— is a clue to what type of JRA a person has.

Pauciarticular JRA

"Pauci" means "few," and those who get this type of JRA have only a few joints—usually fewer than five—affected by the disease. These joints tend to be in the legs. Sometimes eyes can become inflamed as well. This condition, known as iritis, can often be detected only by an ophthalmologist (an eye doctor). Iritis usually lasts only for a few weeks or months. If discovered early, it can be easily treated with eye drops. This type of JRA most often appears in girls under the age of ten.

Most kids with pauciarticular JRA have no sign of arthritis after a few years. However, some later develop polyarticular JRA.

Polyarticular JRA

"Poly" means "many," and this more serious type of JRA affects many joints at once—at least five. More girls than boys are affected, and the onset appears at a later age. In some instances, this is actually an adult form of rheumatoid arthritis that begins earlier than usual.

The onset of one or more inflamed joints can be sudden or gradual. Other early signs are enlarged lymph nodes (particularly under the arms) and subcutaneous nodules (movable but painless lumps under the skin, usually located around the elbows, wrists, ankles, or feet). Although they might appear and disappear over a few months, these symptoms are harmless.

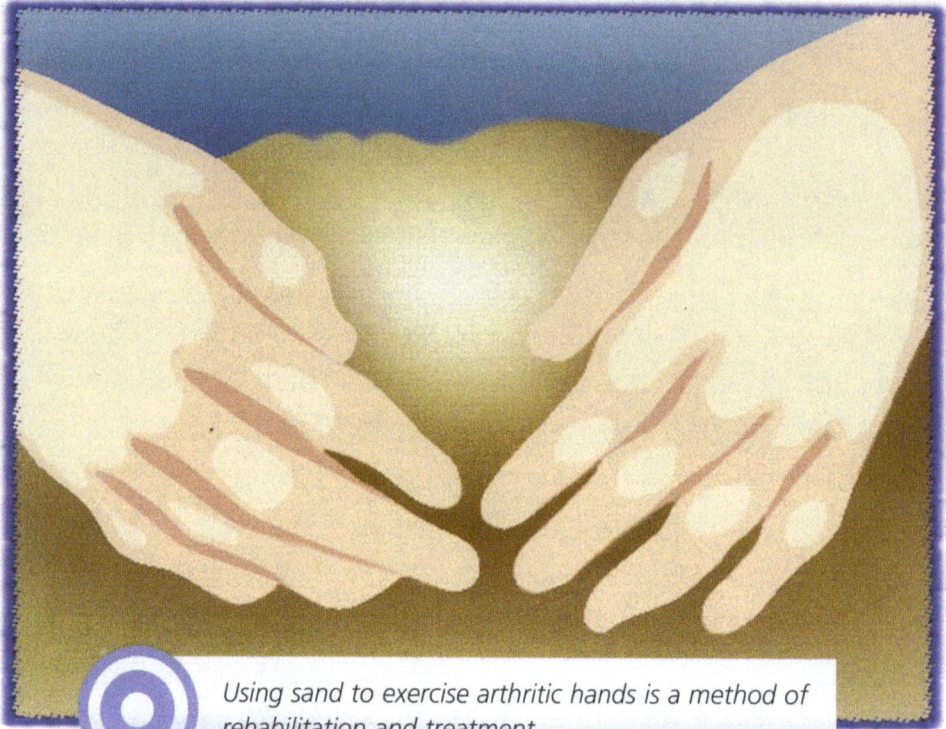

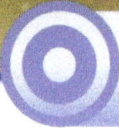

Using sand to exercise arthritic hands is a method of rehabilitation and treatment.

Because of the number of joints involved, this type of JRA is the most severe and potentially destructive. Serious injury to joints, bones, and cartilage, as well as the loss of motion in joints, are a great risk. This is why early and aggressive treatment with physical therapy and medicine are especially important. Although kids with polyarticular JRA are the most likely to experience some loss of motion as well as have their arthritis continue into adulthood, most are able to go to school, get jobs, have families, and live and function on their own.

Systemic JRA

Unlike the other two types of the disease, in which swollen, stiff, and painful joints are the first signs, kids with systemic JRA also experience extremely high fevers (up to 105°F) and a strange, splotchy pink rash. Both the fevers and the rash come and go daily, sometimes twice a day. They never last for more than a few weeks at a time. The rheumatoidal rash is one of the strangest things ever seen. You can literally watch it move around a body in a matter of minutes. Usually smooth and salmon-colored, it has distinct irregular borders and a pale center. It can range in size from a small button to a baseball.

Systemic JRA also attacks a child's internal organs. The sac around the heart can fill up with fluid. The liver, spleen, and lymph nodes often swell up. Kidneys and blood cells are affected, too. However, with proper medical attention, these inflammations rarely cause serious problems.

The fevers and rashes typical of systemic JRA rarely last for more than five years, and they don't cause any damage to the body. Fevers and rashes usually accompany flares of arthritis, but the fever can be easily controlled with medication. The arthritis involved can be either pauciarticular or polyarticular.

Chapter 2

Symptoms and Diagnosis

Symptoms are physical signs that your body isn't working properly. A symptom can affect the way you look, function, and feel. Most symptoms indicate a type of sickness or disease. In the previous chapter, we looked at the symptoms that indicate the onset of the three types of JRA. In all cases, the main symptom is inflammation—redness, heat, and swelling accompanied by pain—in the joints. Stiffness in the joints, particularly in the morning or during cold, damp weather, is common. When a joint is very stiff, it is almost impossible to move it. This immobility can last for ten minutes or ten hours. Furthermore, certain types of JRA have specific symptoms such as iritis, spiking fevers, or the rheumatoidal rash. These symptoms are all indications that you may have JRA.

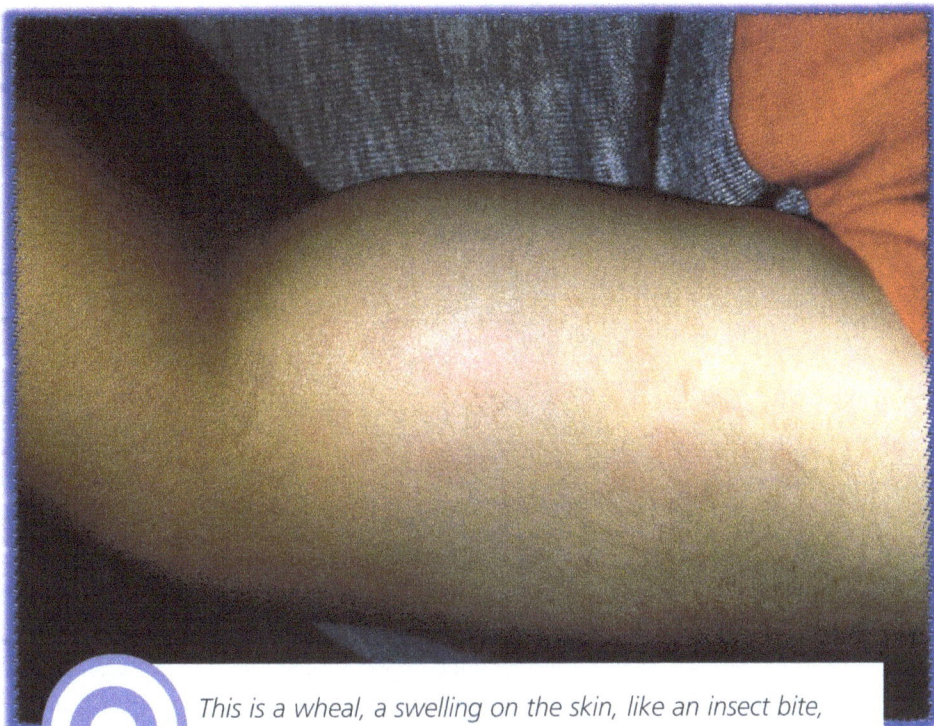

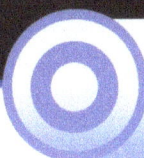

This is a wheal, a swelling on the skin, like an insect bite, that usually itches or burns. Wheals can accompany JRA.

Whatever you do, don't pretend that your symptoms don't exist or that they will go away on their own. Too often, young people who experience JRA symptoms first pretend that nothing is wrong with them. They might feel afraid and hope that the symptoms will just disappear. However, controlling JRA depends on being diagnosed and treated as quickly as possible. If you experience any of the symptoms described earlier, tell your parents or a close relative and get medical attention immediately.

Diagnosis

A diagnosis is the identification of a disease or condition based on exams and tests. Even if you have the classic symptoms of JRA, a diagnosis is important to know the nature and seriousness of the disease and to plan a treatment strategy.

Other diseases may have symptoms similar to those of JRA. These include certain infections, tumors, musculoskeletal conditions, lupus, leukemia, fibromyalgia, and other rare rheumatic diseases. Thorough testing is necessary to make sure that you really do have JRA and not another condition.

Testing

I couldn't believe how many tests there were. I missed a lot of school just sitting around in different doctors' waiting rooms. I can't even remember how many times the nurses asked for blood or urine samples. Luckily, the technicians are really smooth at drawing blood. I barely felt the needles.

The worst thing is that there's no one test that can tell you if you have JRA. I was going nuts not knowing what was happening to me. I was always really athletic and suddenly it was all taken away from me. Not knowing what was going on with my body was almost worse than the pain. Even after I was diagnosed with JRA, my doctor didn't know when, or even if, I would get better. However, know-ing that 80 percent of young people with the condition grow up to lead normal lives made me determined to be one of them.

—Paul

To receive a diagnosis, you must often see several types of doctors and undergo many examinations and tests. These also allow specialists to determine the seri-ousness of your JRA and to detect any complications.

After giving the doctor your family history (perhaps there are cases of arthritis or rheumatism in your family) and your personal medical history, you will need to have a complete physical examination. The doctor will pay special attention to your joints and also look for rashes, lumps under the skin, or swollen lymph nodes.

X rays will reveal the condition of your joints and bones and whether you have any fractures, tumors, or infections. They can also reveal inflamed internal organs such as your liver or kidneys. Sometimes a joint/bone scan is necessary. This is done by injecting radioactive fluid into your joints and then checking for inflammation.

Many types of laboratory tests are often necessary. Joint and tissue fluids can be examined for infections or inflammation. Blood tests can reveal many things, including the presence of an RF factor, a special type of antibody that is present in many young people with

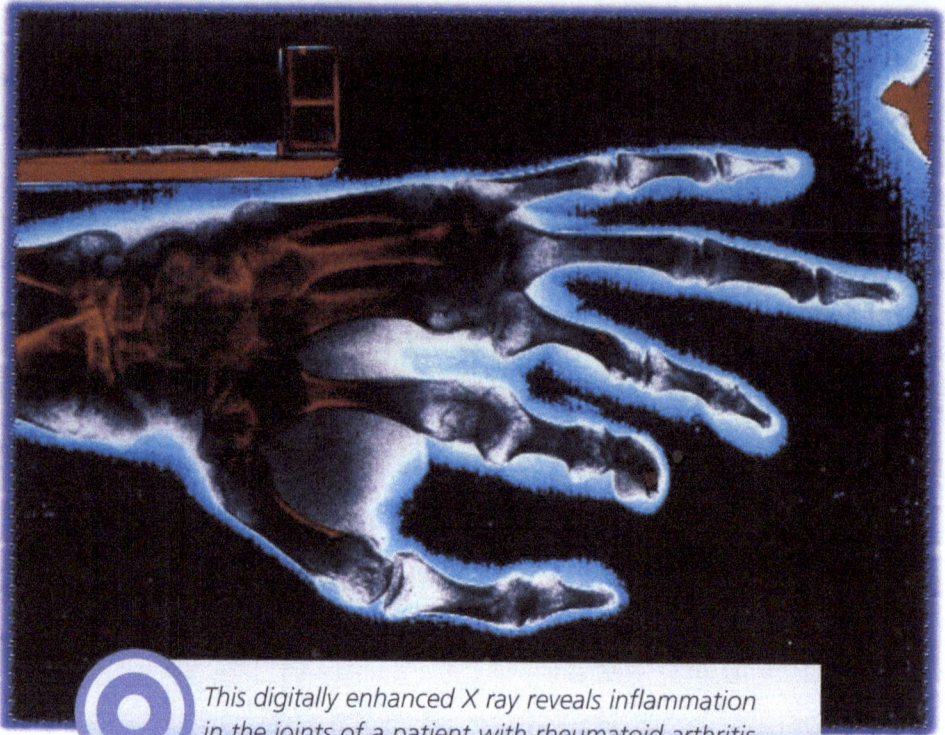

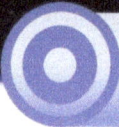

This digitally enhanced X ray reveals inflammation in the joints of a patient with rheumatoid arthritis.

polyarticular JRA, as well as most adults with arthritis. They might also reveal a decrease in red blood cells that could lead to anemia (which leaves you feeling weak and tired)—another symptom of systemic JRA. Both blood and urine tests show how organs such as the lungs and kidneys are working. They also help rule out the possibility of other diseases.

Taking an ultrasound of your heart, known as an echocardiogram, allows doctors to see if there is a sac of fluid around your heart, which is a symptom of systemic JRA. Seeing an ophthalmologist is important, too. Often only he or she can detect the presence of iritis.

Chapter 3

Treatment

For a long time it was thought that juvenile arthritis didn't exist. Even when experts did finally admit that young people could get rheumatoid arthritis, they believed that nothing much could be done to treat it. It was all too common to simply send a child to bed with some aspirin for the pain and inflammation. Since moving around proved difficult and painful, kids with JRA stayed in bed for weeks, months, or even longer periods of time. Not moving at all, however, didn't lessen the inflammation of their joints. Instead, they swelled up even more and often destroyed surrounding muscles and bones. Lack of exercise caused muscles to atrophy, or waste away, to the point of being useless.

These kids ended up in wheelchairs or confined to their homes or hospitals, where they were completely dependent on nurses or family members. Unable to go to school, play outside, or have a social life, such kids were often depressed and insecure. This kind of isolated existence did not equip them to deal with the challenges of a normal life. Some serious cases were confined to bed, and sometimes placed in body casts, until they were fully grown. At this point, their damaged joints could be replaced, through surgery, with artificial ones. Even with replacements, though, their bodies were often so crippled that many sufferers were confined to wheelchairs for life. And a lifetime of arthritis had left them so immobile that leading a "normal" life was sometimes impossible.

Knowledge about and treatment of JRA have come a long way in a short time. With proper treatment, it is increasingly possible for kids with JRA to not only lead full lives as children and teenagers but as adults as well.

Teamwork

Because JRA can affect many joints and body parts, it is difficult for one doctor to care for a patient. Often he or she simply doesn't possess knowledge in so many different fields. And doctors aren't only concerned with treating the arthritis—they want to treat the whole child. The best way to do this is by having a coordinated group of specialists working together. This group is known as the

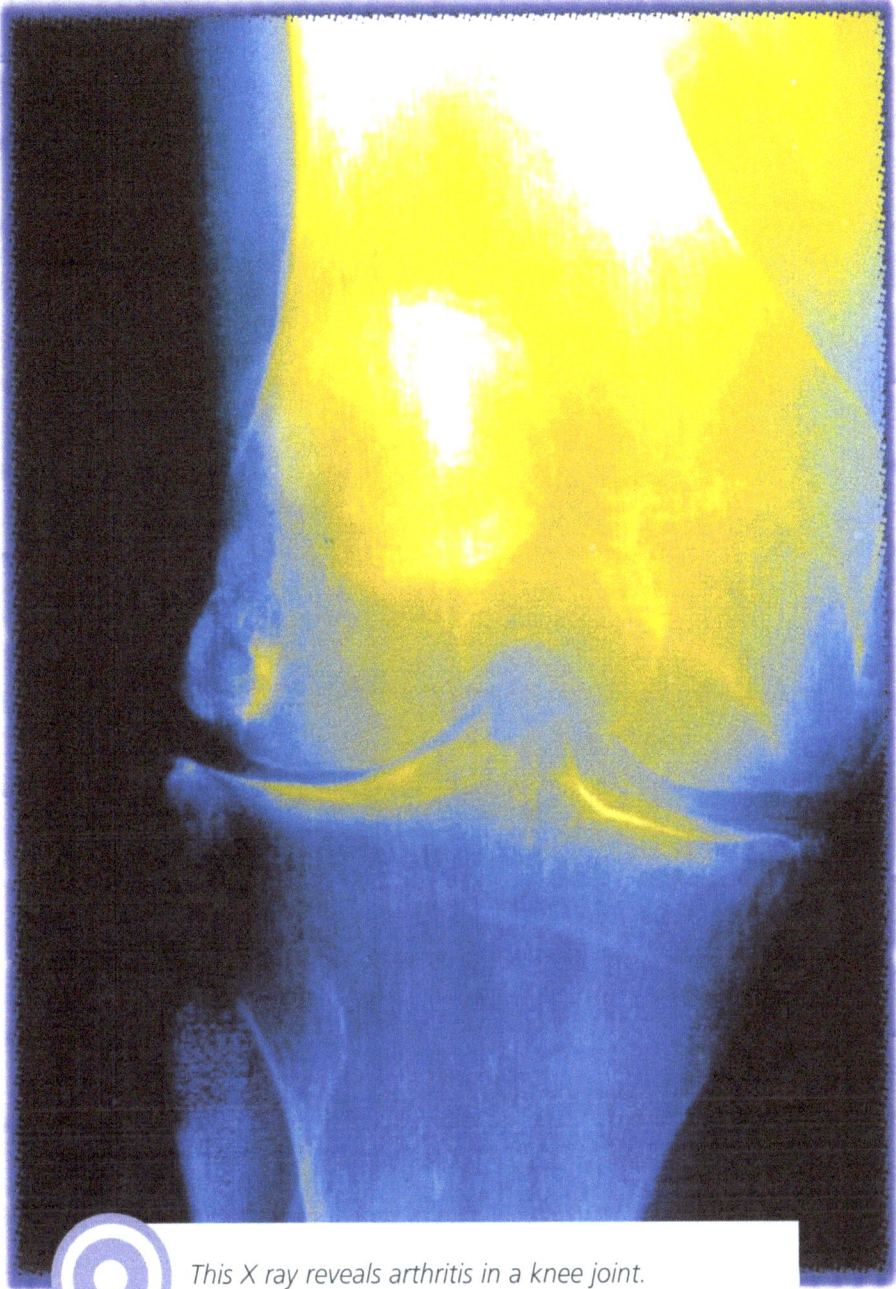

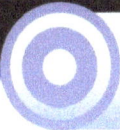

This X ray reveals arthritis in a knee joint.

pediatric rheumatology team. Such teams can be found in the growing number of pediatric rheumatology centers across North America. Pediatric doctors specialize in diseases that affect children and teens. In general, the following specialists are members of a pediatric rheumatology team:

Pediatric Rheumatologist

A pediatric rheumatologist specializes in treating young people with arthritic and rheumatic conditions. These diseases often affect kids, whose bodies are still growing, differently than adults. The pediatrician you see will do your medical and family history and physical examination. After giving you and your family a diagnosis, he or she will make up a plan based on your needs.

Nurse

A nurse is often the team coordinator who serves as a go-between for the other medical specialists, the patient, and the family. Specialists are often very busy. The nurse can monitor you and help educate you and your family. The nurse is usually the one who does blood tests, schedules appointments with specialists, and explains doctors' sometimes complicated jargon to patients and families. You can usually call the team nurse with any problems or questions. He or she will get in touch with the necessary specialist and get back to you.

Physical Therapist

The physical therapist examines your muscles and joints to see how they are working. The examination concludes with a functional assessment. This is a list of the tasks that you can and cannot do based on the severity of your JRA and the joints affected at a given moment. Assessments are ongoing since your condition might change, grow worse, or improve over time. Once an assessment is made, together with other diagnoses and opinions, the therapist can design and monitor an exercise program for you that works your joints.

He or she should also make up a general exercise program as well. A general exercise program is for the entire body—to maintain overall health. It is important not only to keep your joints strong and mobile, but to make sure your whole body is physically fit.

Social Worker

A social worker can help deal with problems that might emerge in your family or at school. Social workers have experience in counseling families. Sometimes parents might feel stressed or afraid. Brothers and sisters might feel left out. Social workers can also talk to teachers and principals and help enforce programs that allow you to continue being educated at school as much as possible. They are also great sources of information when looking for community support programs.

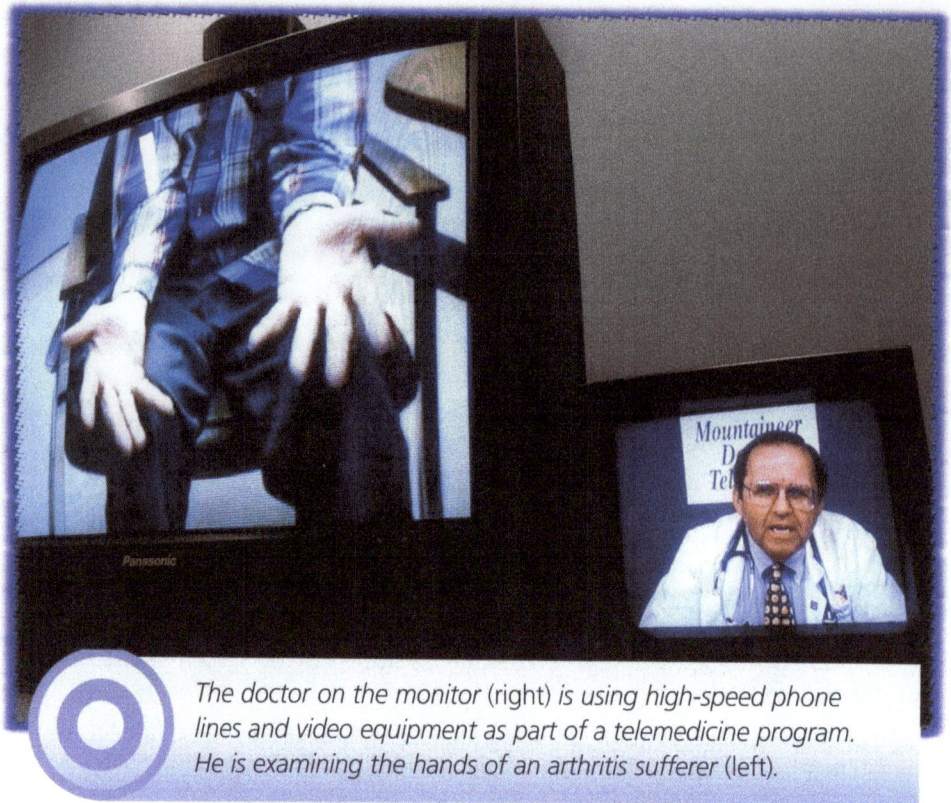

The doctor on the monitor (right) is using high-speed phone lines and video equipment as part of a telemedicine program. He is examining the hands of an arthritis sufferer (left).

Educator

JRA is a complex disease, and an important part of battling it successfully is knowing and understanding as much as possible about it. Many centers have educators who will explain the disease and its effects to you and your family. The educator can talk about treatments, drugs (and their side effects), and new medical breakthroughs. Nurses often assume the role of educator.

Nutritionist

Weight loss and growth problems experienced by kids with JRA are due more to poor nutrition than to the disease itself. The fact is that most Americans don't eat healthful diets. If you have JRA, a well-balanced diet is essential to keeping strong. And if the disease or side effects from medication are affecting your appetite, you will need advice on special diets. All of these tasks are the job of a nutritionist.

Working with the Results: Creating a Plan

Once all tests are carried out and a complete diagnosis has been made, the team members share their results with each other. Then they discuss them with you and your parents. Together you create a plan of attack. This includes medication, physical therapy, nutrition, family support, school and other community services, and, if needed, psychological counseling. The team should also communicate the diagnosis and plan to your family doctor or pediatrician. He or she is the one who will continue caring for you on an ongoing basis.

The effects of JRA can be very complex. They can affect every aspect of your life and the rest of your family members, too. That's why it is so good to have a team of specialists who know the ropes and can help you and your family cope. They can coordinate treatment with your family doctor or pediatrician, with other doctors (ophthalmologists, orthopedic surgeons, and adult rheumatologists, for instance), and with other health professionals (including psychologists and dentists). The specialists can also guide you and your family to school and community resources that can help you lead as full a life as possible.

Chapter 4

Fighting Back

Although there is no cure for JRA, there are ways of fighting the disease to keep it under control as much as possible. There are two main weapons used to battle JRA: prescribed medication and physical therapy.

Medication

The choice of drugs for young people with JRA is similar to those used for adult arthritis. Doses depend on a child's size and age as well as the nature and severity of the disease. Medication can be changed frequently, depending on how the disease advances. However, drugs that work for one person might not work for another. Or they might work for a while and then gradually—or even overnight—lose effect. Other drugs might work well but may have serious side effects. If the side effects are severe, it's a good idea to look for another type of medication. For these reasons, finding a drug that works is often a long, drawn-out process of elimination.

There are two types of drugs used to treat JRA: nonsteroidal anti-inflammatory drugs and second-line drugs.

Nonsteroidal Anti-Inflammatory Drugs (NSAIDs)

One of the most traditional drugs used to fight inflammation is aspirin. Aspirin is a nonsteroidal anti-inflammatory drug that fights inflammation as well as fever. However, many kids with JRA take aspirin in large doses over long periods. In some cases, the aspirin eats away at their livers and kidneys. The damage can be permanent.

When I was first diagnosed with JRA, I had thirty-nine joints inflamed and I was taking sixteen baby aspirins a day. It really worked wonders. In the early stages, I was going into the rheumatology center every week for blood tests. After five months, the doctor found that the aspirin was causing damage to my liver. A day after I stopped taking it, I was in so much pain that I just lay in bed crying. I couldn't even stand to be touched. It took a week for the aspirin to wash completely out of my system. Then the doctors had to start testing new medication that could control my symptoms without such serious side effects. Over a seven-year period, I took fifteen different medications. Some worked really well—for a while. Others didn't work at all.

—Rosa

Ibuprofen, naprosen (also known as naproxen), and relafen are other common NSAIDs used to fight swelling, redness, pain, and fever. They tend to be less destructive on the internal organs than aspirin. Common brands of ibuprofen include Advil, Motrin, Nuprin, and Rufen.

In most cases of JRA, these anti-inflammatory drugs are the first to be prescribed since they are the fastest and the safest. Of course, fast means that it takes them a matter of weeks to take effect. During this trial period, doses are low and testing is done to monitor the effects and side effects. In general, 50 percent of kids with JRA respond to the first NSAID they try. Most try two or three before they find the one that works the best for them.

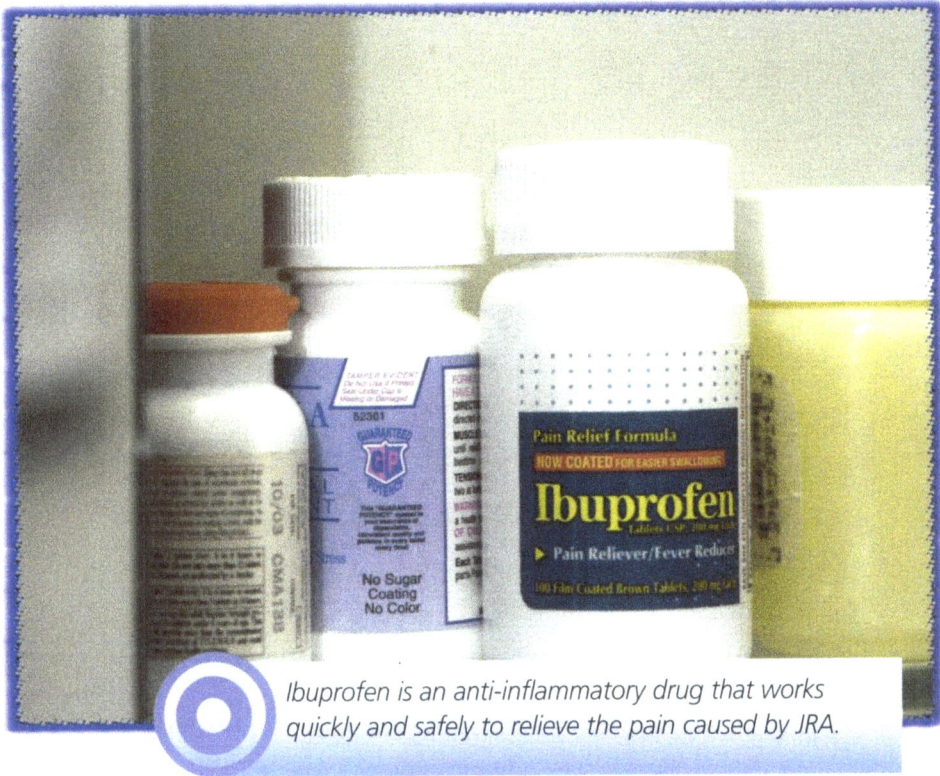

Ibuprofen is an anti-inflammatory drug that works quickly and safely to relieve the pain caused by JRA.

Second-Line Drugs

If after trying various NSAIDs, your JRA hasn't improved or is growing worse, second-line drugs will be added to your medication program. There are many different kinds of these drugs. The most widely used and efficient is methotrexate. Sulfasalazine, hydroxychloroquine, and penicillamine are also common. Some of these drugs must be taken for months before they have an effect. They are all strong anti-inflammatory drugs.

One of the fastest acting second-line drugs that gets the best results is cortisone. It is also the most potentially dangerous. Although cortisone is a steroid, it is not similar to the male hormone steroids taken by athletes and body-builders who want to bulk up. Instead, it suppresses the immune system in order to stop inflammation.

Initially, taking cortisone can produce miraculous effects. Within days, a child confined to bed who is crying out in pain can be outside running around without any soreness or stiffness. The problem is that in order to maintain these results, doses must be continuously increased. At a certain point, cortisone not only becomes ineffective, but it can create serious side effects. The most dangerous side effect in children is that it can stop their bodies from growing. Reducing the dosage can cause symptoms to return even worse than before.

Cortisone is often used as a last resort in serious cases. Yet when prescribed in small doses and carefully monitored, it can be a safe and effective way of reducing damage to your body.

Side Effects

Side effects depend on the person taking the drugs, the amount or dose of the drug, and the combination of different medications. Although NSAIDs have many possible side effects, few cause major problems. Some of the most common side effects are nausea, abdominal pain, vomiting, diarrhea, headaches, and drowsiness.

With second-line drugs, side effects can be more severe. Cortisone is probably the most dangerous of these drugs. It can not only stunt growth but can cause an increased appetite, which in turn leads to weight gain. It can also lead to fluid retention, which not only causes swelling but high blood pressure as well. Other side effects include weakening of the bones and mood swings.

Alternative Treatments

Sometimes young people try alternative treatments for JRA. Alternative treatments are those not usually pre-scribed by doctors. There are thousands of herbs, medi-cines, foods, and devices (such as copper bracelets) that are believed to help those with JRA feel better. Most are harmless, but a few are dangerous. None have been proven to cure JRA. Although a few might momentarily relieve symptoms, taking them along with your pre-scribed medicines could cause many problems and put your treatment—and your body—at risk.

Physical Therapy

Along with drug therapy, physical therapy is one of the most important ways of ensuring that you have as much mobility as possible. Physical therapy consists of various types of exercise and heat treatments that strengthen muscles, stretch muscles that have stiffened, and allow you to maintain the motion of your joints.

Exercises

Helpful exercises include those that are designed and/or monitored by a trained physical therapist. They may include unstructured activities such as swimming, rowing, or even playing with clay. Activities in water are especially good. A full exercise program usually consists of the following types of exercise:

- **Active—Series of knee-bends, sit-ups, and toe-touches are great for building up strength and endurance.**

- **Active assistive—When somebody assists or helps you to do the above type of exercise.**

- **Active resistant—Pushing or flexing muscles against a resisting object (a wall or a person's hand) helps keep them strong.**

- **Passive—When your pain is so great that you can't move, another person can extend and flex your joints (such as knees or hips) in order to preserve some movement.**

- **Aerobic—Using treadmills, rowing, climbing stairs, and walking are all good for increasing endurance. The best aerobic exercise of all is swimming.**

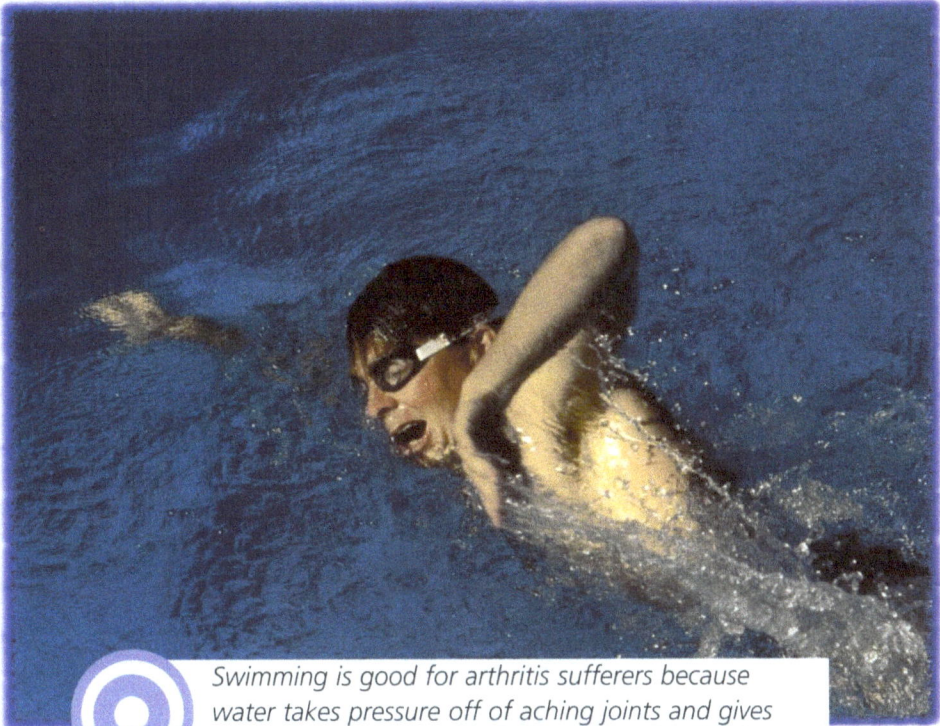

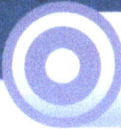

Swimming is good for arthritis sufferers because water takes pressure off of aching joints and gives people the feeling of being weightless.

I love being in the water. I imagine it's the way astronauts feel when they're floating around in space. I try to use the pool at the local YWCA at least every other day, and the local Arthritis Foundation in our town has a special aquatic program where I can do exercises with other kids who have JRA. Being in the water makes me feel so free. It takes all the pressure off my joints. I can do so many things in the pool that I can't do on dry land.

When I'm down or stressed or in a lot of pain, there's nothing like a long, hot bath. And days when I wake up really stiff and worried that I won't make it down the stairs, let alone get to school, a long, hot shower is sometimes the best thing to get me going.

—*Jill*

Heat Treatment

Heat relaxes muscles and allows you to move your joints with more ease. Moist heat generally works better than dry heat. The easiest access to moist heat is a hot bath or shower. Other types of moist heat are heated swimming pools, hot tubs, steam rooms, and hot packs. All these can help you get going in the morning when your joints are stiff. Before or during exercises, moist heat treatment can reduce pain and muscle spasms, making it easier to complete your physical therapy.

Hot packs are useful when a specific joint or muscle, such as the knee or shoulder, is acting up. An easy way to make a hot pack is to moisten a towel and heat it up in a microwave oven. Another good idea is to sleep on a heated waterbed.

Splints, Crutches, and Braces

Splints are used to keep joints in their proper position and to prevent pain. Arm and hand splints are generally

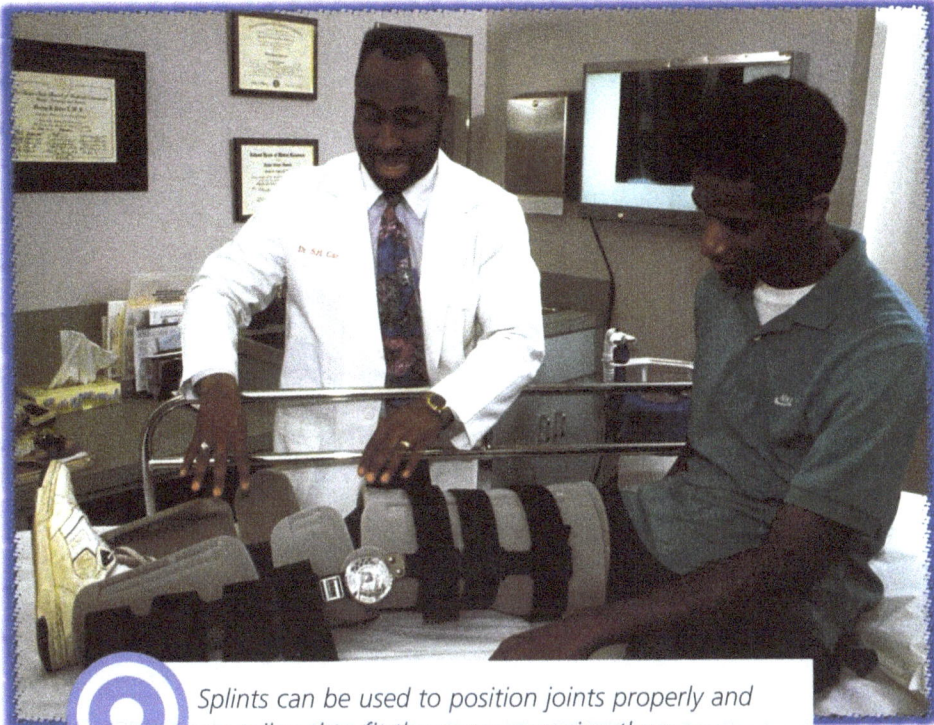

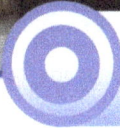

Splints can be used to position joints properly and are tailored to fit the person wearing them.

made from plastic by a physical therapist. Leg splints are made from cast material by an orthopedic specialist. Most splints are worn at night when you are sleeping, since you need to move your joints during the day. However, using a splint during the day can help make getting around easier. Splints are made for each individual. They are adjusted as you grow or as the position of your joints change. Crutches and braces are usually avoided because they can weaken legs and bones. However, sometimes they are essential for kids who truly can't walk.

Surgery

Most kids with JRA will never need surgery. However, in a few severe cases where a great deal of damage or destruction has been caused to joints and surrounding bones, surgery may be the best option. Joints may be operated on to return them to their correct position or to stabilize them. In serious cases, doctors may recommend total joint replacement surgery in which a damaged joint is replaced with an entirely new, artificial one that can last for up to fifteen or twenty years.

Joint replacement surgery is now being performed on kids as young as ten. However, most receive artificial joints at later stages when they are fully grown. Many different types of artificial joints are available, but the most common are hip and knee replacements made out of metal or plastic. Some joints are standard off-the-shelf models while others are tailor-made. Although recuperating from surgery can be a long process with lots of physical therapy, there are few complications involved. Furthermore, kids who could barely move or were in excruciating pain are almost as good as new.

Chapter 5

Coping at School

School is one of the most important aspects of your life. Getting an education and interacting with kids your own age is part of growing up and becoming an adult. Even though you might have JRA, it is essential to stay in school as often and for as long as possible. These days, homebound or in-hospital education with a tutor is rarely needed for more than brief periods of time.

Of course, there are days when simply getting on a bus or walking through the freezing cold to school is a painful challenge. Lugging around heavy books, going up and down stairs to different classrooms, staying seated in one position for an hour, even standing in line at the cafeteria might prove to be very challenging. Yet none of this means that you can't go to school like other kids.

American federal law 94-142 (originally called the Individuals with Disabilities Education Act) guarantees the right of all children to equal education regardless of physical disabilities. This means that if you have JRA, you have the right to the same education as your peers. Under this law, you have the right to special services. These special services can be outlined in an Individualized Education Plan (IEP). An IEP is a study plan developed by you, your parents, school teachers, nurses, principals, and concerned specialists such as your team nurse, social worker, and/or physical therapist. It takes into account what you are and are not able to do because of your condition. And it helps you come up with solutions to problems that would otherwise make it difficult for you to attend classes.

Dear Mr. Galloway,
I have been assigned to your homeroom class. I have arthritis and would like you to know more about me. Although you might not be able to tell by looking, I'm sometimes in a lot of pain. If I'm quiet or distracted, it doesn't mean that I'm not interested in your lesson. Mornings can be difficult because sometimes my joints are very stiff. Sometimes by the end of the day, I can be tired. A lot of the time, however, I feel fine.

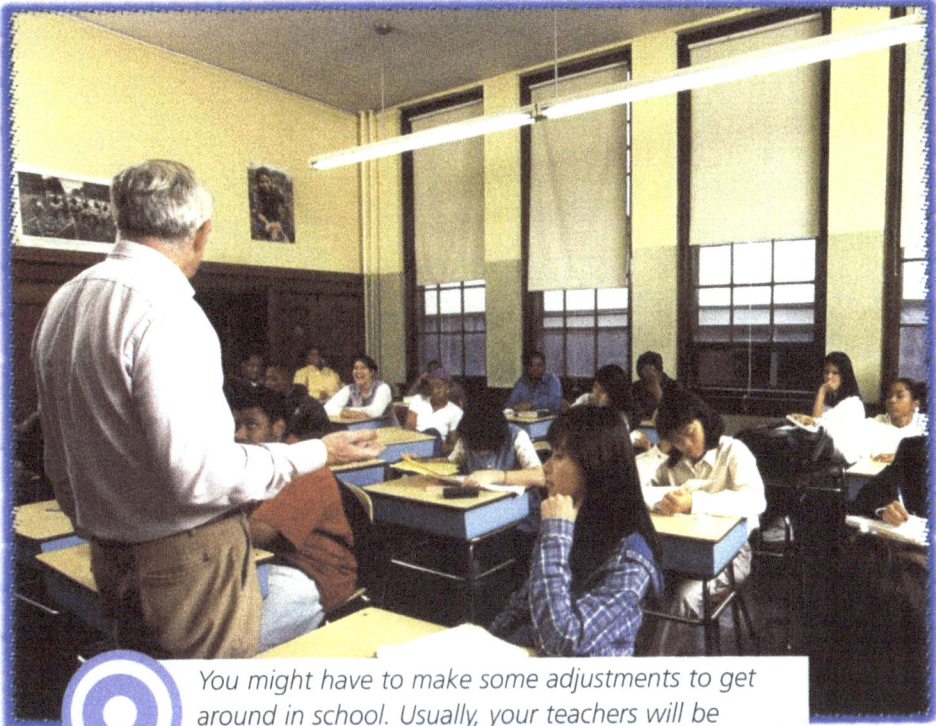

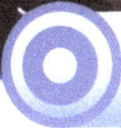

You might have to make some adjustments to get around in school. Usually, your teachers will be willing to work with you.

It's very important for me to be in school as much as possible. I want to be involved as much as I can in all activities. Sometimes, though, we might need to work out special arrangements. I can't always participate in regular playground or athletic programs. I will need to take medication at school and at times I might need to get up in class and stretch my joints. From time to time, I may need to miss school to see my doctor or physical therapist.

I hope you can meet with my parents and me at the beginning of the school year so that we can understand each other better. My parents will keep you informed if there are important changes in my condition that you need to know about.

It would help a lot if you have the same expectations for me that you do for the other kids. I may be slow or awkward, but I can do the same things that other kids can. If I can't finish an assignment on time, please let me take it home instead of excusing me because of my arthritis.

If you have any questions about my condition, please talk to me or my parents.

Sincerely,

Rob

Many teachers aren't aware of JRA, and many are overworked and may have trouble concentrating on the individual needs of so many students. Because of this, communication—between you, your family, your doctors, and your school—is really important. Sometimes you might not even need to draw up an IEP. Getting together and working out an informal agreement might be enough. The key is good communication and the ability to work together.

For instance, it may be hard for you to stay seated without moving for a long time. Yet your teacher might find that it disrupts the class to have you stand up and stretch. Choosing you to erase the boards or hand out papers might be a good compromise for both of you. Similarly, it might be hard for you to run the bases during a baseball game, but that doesn't mean you have to sit on the sidelines. Ask your physical education instructor if another player can be a designated runner and go around the bases after you pop a homer.

From scheduling your classes close together and keeping sets of heavy textbooks both at home and at school to scheduling rest periods at the nurse's office and substituting a written exam with an oral one, there are many solutions to the problems you might face as a student with JRA.

Just remember that you have a right to the same education as every other person, and that right is protected by law. To help you learn your rights, you and your parents should definitely take a look at "Educational Rights for Children with Arthritis: A Manual for Parents," published by the American Juvenile Arthritis Organization (AJAO) of the Arthritis Foundation.

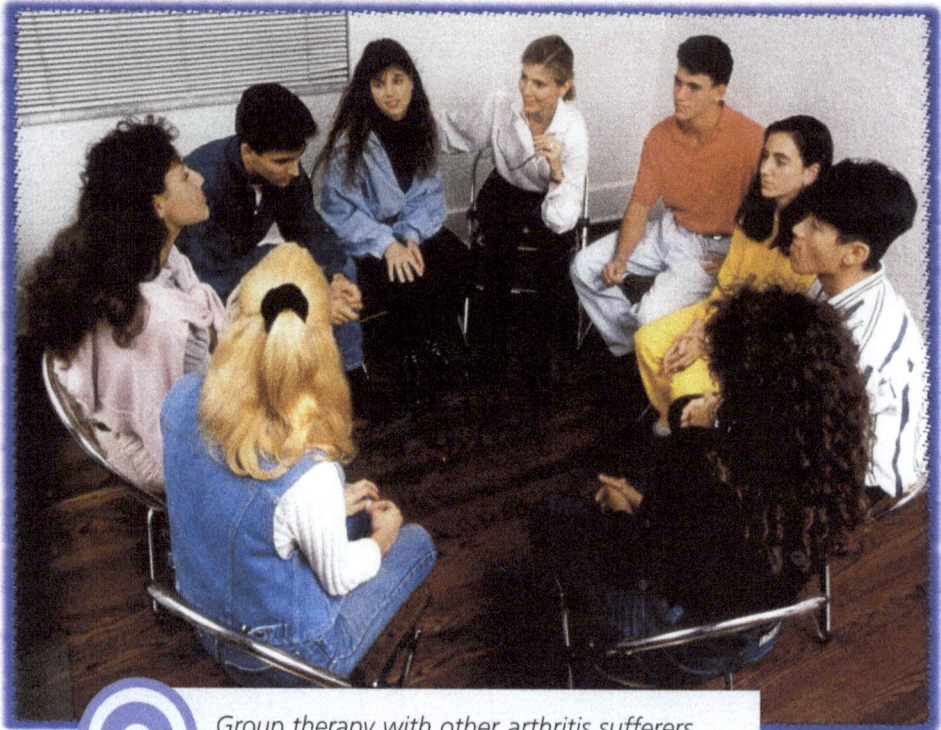

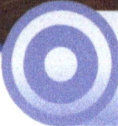

Group therapy with other arthritis sufferers your age can help you cope with your illness.

You and Your Peers

When growing up, nobody likes to feel different from the rest of the group. It's hard for anyone to go through adolescence. Just imagine how much more complicated life is if you're a teen with JRA. As mentioned earlier, a lot of kids with JRA try to hide their condition, especially if it's not so severe. They're afraid of being seen as different or disabled. They fear being excluded or treated differently from other kids.

Unfortunately, you can't pretend that you don't have JRA and you won't be able to continually fake that nothing's wrong. Sure, there will be moments when you feel fine and you can do everything any kid can do. But other times, a flare will sneak up on you. You'll need your friends' support, understanding, and sometimes their help. Hiding the fact that you have JRA doesn't help anybody: neither you nor your friends nor the treatment of the disease. It will create stress and unhappiness for you and leave your friends feeling puzzled and even excluded.

It is nobody's fault you have JRA—especially not your own—and the disease is nothing to be ashamed of. In fact, dealing with it openly and honestly and trying to live a full life in spite of it is courageous. Most friends and peers will respect and admire you all the more if you adopt this attitude.

People fear what they don't understand. So instead of pretending that you don't have JRA, let your friends and classmates know about the disease up front. They might not understand why one minute you're lobbing around a volleyball with them and the next minute you have to lie down in the bleachers. Try educating them. Explain how the disease works and why you feel the way you do.

Furthermore, get involved and stay involved. If you can't play basketball anymore, what about trying to become the team's manager or its official photographer?

Chapter 6

Coping at Home

Juvenile arthritis will not only change your life but the lives of your family members as well. It can at times be tough to deal with, so it's extremely important to be patient, open, and honest.

I was twelve when I first starting having problems with my knees. They were really sore, and I found it hard to walk. My dad thought I was just out of shape. When I told him I didn't think I could play football anymore, he told me I was a quitter. When my knee went back to normal after a few weeks, he said that this was proof I had been faking. He even had me wondering if I'd made everything up. But then a year later, the pain and swelling returned. And this time in my toes and hips as well. My dad didn't believe me, but when it got so bad I couldn't walk, my mom insisted on taking me to a pediatric rheumatologist.

When I was finally diagnosed with JRA, things were really bad at home. My mom cried all the time and fussed over me. She wouldn't let me do anything for fear I would fall down and break my bones. Meanwhile, my dad grew really distant. He had always wanted me to play football. Now that seemed next to impossible.

—Fernando

You and Your Parents

It's very difficult for parents to see their children suffering. Some parents might refuse to accept that you have JRA or that it is as severe as doctors say. They may try to go on as if nothing is wrong and not take your symptoms and complaints seriously. They might initially feel shock and outrage that their healthy son or daughter has come down with a chronic, complicated condition with no cure. They might even feel guilty and blame themselves if their family has a history of arthritic or rheumatic problems.

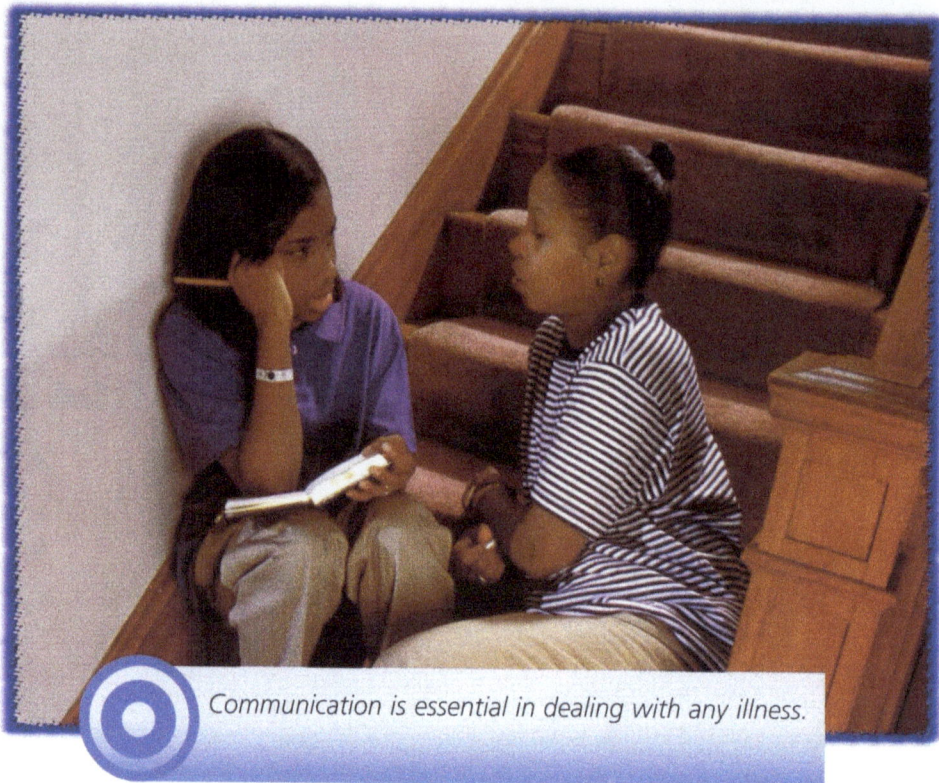

Communication is essential in dealing with any illness.

Some parents may become overprotective. They'll worry about you—sometimes too much. They might order your siblings to do all the household chores or not let you go out with your friends, fearing that these activities will prove too difficult for you. It's up to you to let them know that, even if it's hard, you want to lead as normal a life as possible. Of course, nobody likes washing dishes or emptying the garbage. However, using your condition as an excuse to get out of doing things that you simply don't feel like doing would be dishonest.

Things can be particularly scary following the onset of JRA. Neither you nor your parents know what is going on with your body. And even the best medical experts can't predict how long JRA will last, how it will progress, and what treatments will or won't work. This can create a lot of fear and frustration for everybody.

Feeling powerless might cause your mother or father to become obsessed with taking care of you and fighting your disease. It is wonderful to have love and support, and you will obviously need to rely on your parents much more now than before you had JRA. However, if you feel that your parents have become obsessed with your condition, that they are depressed and exhausted, or that they no longer go out with friends or each other, talk to them. Tell them that in order for them to help you and the rest of your family, they need to be healthy. Part of being healthy is having a balanced life with some time to take care of themselves.

Your parents should know all about JRA, what you're going through now, and what you (and they) might have to deal with in the future. This means becoming knowledgeable about the disease and discussing all diagnoses, tests, and treatment options. Better still, have your parents join a support group for families of kids with JRA. They will encounter both practical help and emotional support. Nobody knows more about dealing with the ups and downs of JRA than other families with JRA.

You and Your Siblings

It is equally important that your brothers and/or sisters learn as much as possible about JRA and how they can help you. Not telling them about the disease can leave them feeling left out. Obviously, it is easier for older siblings to understand this complicated disease. However, keeping younger kids in the dark by not talking about issues such as pain and immobility is often much scarier than carefully explaining as many facts as possible.

It may be hard for your siblings to deal with the changes in family life caused by JRA. Some siblings might feel guilty that they can't take away your pain. They might wonder why you have arthritis instead of them. Perhaps they will be afraid—of your symptoms growing worse, or even that they might get arthritis. Sadness is common. So is jealousy and resentment.

Your parents will need to devote more time and attention, and spend more money on you than before. Even older kids who understand the reasons for this might be angry or jealous that their parents don't have time for them. Faced with your parents' increased responsibilities and your physical limitations, your siblings might have to pitch in a lot more at home. Although most siblings will actually find relief in being able to help out, they could also feel resentful. They might take this anger out on your parents—or even on you.

PRACTICAL HELP FROM THE ARTHRITIS FOUNDATION

Diet and Your Arthritis

PRACTICAL HELP FROM THE ARTHRITIS FOUNDATION

When Your Student Has Arthritis
A Guide For Teachers

PRACTICAL HELP FROM THE ARTHRITIS FOUNDATION

Aspirin and Other NSAIDs

PRACTICAL HELP FROM THE ARTHRITIS FOUNDATION

Decision Making for Teenagers with Arthritis

ARTHRITIS FOUNDATION®
Take Control. We Can Help™

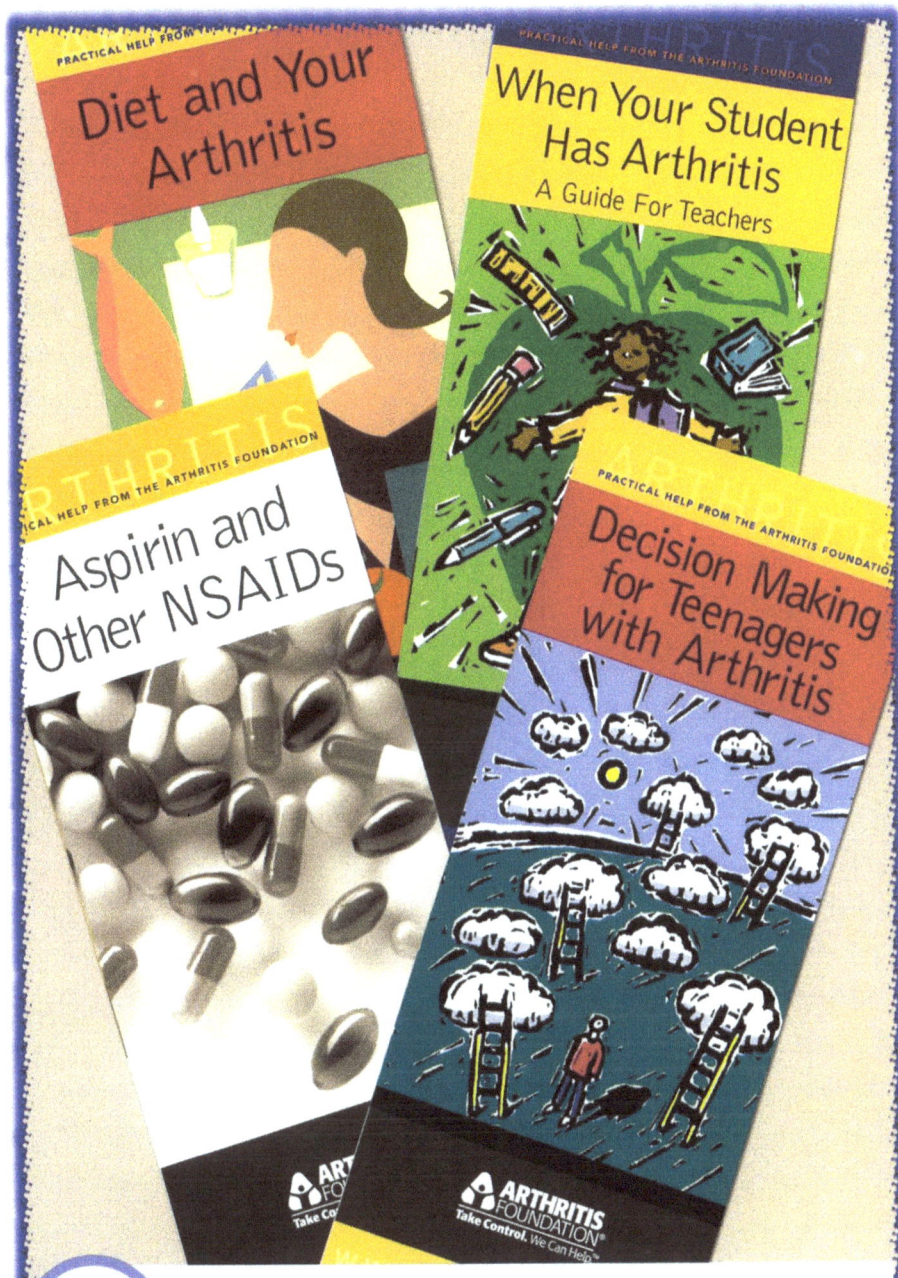

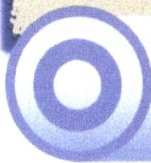

The Arthritis Foundation is the only national organization that supports those with arthritis and related conditions. It offers resources for parents and teens living with juvenile arthritis.

Because these and other family problems are so common, most pediatric rheumatoid arthritis teams include a social worker. This is a professional with experience in counseling JRA families and helping them work through their problems. When problems become really difficult, your social worker, doctor, or local arthritis support group can recommend a good psychologist that offers both individual and family therapy.

When I think back to when I was first diagnosed with JRA, I'm amazed at how far I've come. For a long time, it all seemed so hopeless: the medications that didn't work, the splints I had to wear, the fear I'd end up in a wheelchair or always be in pain.

But today, ten years later, I just graduated from college and have begun my first job. I work at a physical therapy clinic where I am in charge of the aquatics fitness program. Many kids I work with have JRA. Recently, I also moved in with my boyfriend of two years. He is a wonderful guy who is supportive on my bad days.

I am happy to say that the bad days are infrequent. Two years ago, I began seeing a good adult rheumatologist with whom I have a great relationship. I still take my medication every day. I also exercise every other day: swimming, using the treadmill, and lifting weights. I do a lot of manual therapy, too. Even though my wrists, hands, and shoulders still sometimes become inflamed, my hips and knees almost never act up. Two years ago, I had surgery on my big left toe with fusion and a screw at DIP. Since then I've had no problems at all.

I'm so glad I never gave up. I never let the pain take over my life. Instead, I tried to incorporate the pain into my life. And when things got tough, I had a lot of support. Joining the American Juvenile Arthritis Organization was a great idea—not only for me but for my parents, too. I've remained close with many of the friends I made.

I still go to Arthritis Foundation meetings. I like to keep up with new research and treatments— for my own sake and for that of the kids I work with. It's incredible how far we've come in fighting JRA in the last ten years. With continued research, education, and public awareness, I'm sure that the fight can only get easier.

—Miranda

Glossary

arthritis Inflammation of the joints, characterized by redness, swelling, heat, and pain.

atrophy A wasting away of a body part, such as a muscle, due to lack of use.

autoimmune When the body's immune system attacks the body.

cartilage Smooth, protective tissue that lines the ends of the bones within a joint.

diagnosis Identification of the specific disease responsible for causing symptoms based on medical tests and exams.

flare When a disease begins acting up or when symptoms return after a remission.

Individualized Education Plan (IEP) A written plan that outlines the special education and related services provided for an individual patient's needs.

inflammation The body's response to injury or infection. Usually protective, it is characterized by redness, swelling, heat, and pain.

iritis Inflammation of the iris, the colored part of the eye.

joint An area of the body where two bones meet, usually to allow movement.

ophthalmologist A doctor who specializes in diagnosis and treatment of eye diseases.

orthopedic surgeon A doctor who performs surgery to repair bone or joint damage.

pediatrician A doctor who specializes in treating children and adolescents.

remission A period in which all of a disease's symptoms disappear.

second-line drug A powerful drug that may slow down or affect the course of arthritis.

splint A device used to keep joints in position and relieve pain.

symptom A physical sign that indicates a medical condition or disease.

tendon A thick band of tissue that connects a muscle to a bone.

ultrasound The use of sound waves to produce an image of internal organs.

X ray An image of a bone or other body organ made with radiation.

Where to Go for Help

In the United States

American Academy of Orthopaedic Surgeons
6300 North River Road
Rosemont, IL 60018-4262
(800) 346-AAOS (2267) or (847) 823-7186
Web site: http://www.aaos.org

American College of Rheumatology
1800 Century Place, Suite 250
Atlanta, GA 30345
(404) 633-3777
Web site: http://www.rheumatology.org

Arthritis Foundation and the American Juvenile
   Arthritis Organization (AJAO)
1330 West Peachtree Street
Atlanta, GA 30309
(800) 283-7800 or (404) 965-7514
Web site: http://www.arthritis.org

Arthritis National Research Foundation
200 Oceangate, Suite 400
Long Beach, CA 90802
(800) 588-CURE (2873)
Web site: http://www.curearthritis.org

Federation for Children with Special Needs
1135 Tremont Street, Suite 420
Boston, MA 02120
(800) 331-0688 or (617) 236-7210
Web site: http://www.fcsn.org

National Institute of Arthritis and Musculoskeletal
   and Skin Diseases Information Clearinghouse
National Institutes of Health
1 AMS Circle
Bethesda, MD 20892-3675
(877) 22-NIAMS (226-4267) or
(301) 495-4484
Web site: http://www.niams.nih.gov

In Canada

Canadian Arthritis Network
250 Dundas Street West, Suite 402
Toronto, ON M5G 1X5
(416) 586-4770
Web site: http://www.arthritisnetwork.ca/index.asp

Canadian Arthritis Society (National Office)
393 University Avenue, Suite 1700
Toronto, ON M5G 1E6
(416) 979-7228
Web site: http://www.arthritis.ca

Web Sites

Due to the changing nature of Internet links, the Rosen Publishing Group, Inc., has developed an online list of Web sites related to the subject of this book. This site is updated regularly. Please use this link to access the list:

http://www.rosenlinks.com/ntk/juar/

For Further Reading

Brewer, Earl J., Jr., and Kathy Cochran Angel. *Parenting a Child with Arthritis.* Los Angeles: Lowell House, 1995.

Cook, Allan R. *Arthritis.* Detroit, MI: Omnigraphics, 1999.

Kehret, Peg. *My Brother Made Me Do It.* New York: Minstrel Books, 2000.

Peacock, Judith. *Juvenile Arthritis* (Perspectives on Disease and Illness). Mankato, MN: LifeMatter, 2000.

Tortorica Aldape, Virginia. *Nicole's Story: A Book About a Girl with Juvenile Rheumatoid Arthritis.* Minneapolis, MN: Lerner Publications, 1996.

Tucker, Lori B., M.D., et al. *Your Child with Arthritis: A Family Guide to Caregiving.* Baltimore, MD: Johns Hopkins University Press, 2000.

Bibliography

About.com. "Arthritis." Retrieved September 2001
(http://www.arthritis.about.com).

Arthritis Canada. Retrieved September 2001
(www.arthritis.ca).

Arthritis Foundation and the American Juvenile
Arthritis Organization (AJAO). Retrieved
September 2001 (http://www.arthritis.org).

Brewer, Earl J., Jr., and Kathy Cochran Angel.
Parenting a Child with Arthritis. Los Angeles:
Lowell House, 1995.

Give Rheumatoid Arthritis Children Encouragement
(G.R.A.C.E). Retrieved September 2001
(http://www.fyldecoast.co.uk/grace/grace.htm).

JRA World. "You Never Have to Be Alone." Retrieved
September 2001 (http://jraworld.arthritisinsight.com).

Pediatric Rheumatology Page. Retrieved September
2001 (http://www.goldscout.com).

Index

About the Author
Guy Fall is a freelance journalist and part-time chef.

Photo Credits
Cover, pp. 43, 50 © Kindra Clineff/Index Stock Imagery; p. 2 © LWA/Stephen Welstead/Corbis; p. 8 © Joaquin Palting/Corbis; pp. 11, 12, 16, 19, 22, 46 © Custom Medical; p. 25 © BSIP Agency/ Index Stock Imagery; p. 28 © AP/Wide World Photos; p. 33 by Cindy Reiman; p. 37 © Warren Morgany/Corbis; p. 39 © Bob Daemmrich/The Image Works; p. 53 courtesy of the Arthritis Foundation.

Design
Thomas Forget

Layout
Tahara Hasan